DIY Healing Salves

Tips on How to Make a Herbal Salve + 15 Miracle Recipes!

Table of content

Introduction

I first wish to thank and congratulate you on downloading **"DIY Healing Salves: Tips On How to Make a Herbal Salve and 15 Miracle Recipes!"** It is becoming more and more obvious that more people are losing their attraction to synthetic drugs and are leaning more towards finding herbal medicine to treat their ailments. This of course is not to say that there are many synthetic drugs out there that are life-savers. It is always a good idea to discuss any changes that you want to make as far as your treatments for certain ailments are concerned with your family doctor first.

Unfortunately with many synthetic medications they come with a long list of side-effects that may often end up creating conditions for the patient that are more unpleasant than the original ailment they are supposed to be treating. Often the trouble lies in the abuse of medications when they are taken in dosages that are not safe. Drugs such as Hydrocortisone, that is used in the treatment of many inflammatory conditions such as arthritis, this is destructive to the adrenal glands it can also lead to an unpleasant disorder known as Cushing's syndrome. This condition can lead to weight gain. Basically modern drugs tend to really take their toll on our bodies, along with an unhealthy diet choice is not good for ones health all round, especially with fast foods or pre-packaged foods that are filled with artificial flavors and chemical additives.

In this book you will enjoy a collection of remedies that will gently heal without suppressing symptoms. Herbal remedies are perfectly safe to use when administered in the correct dosages and they come without the bad side-effects.

Chapter 1. How to Obtain Medicinal Herbs

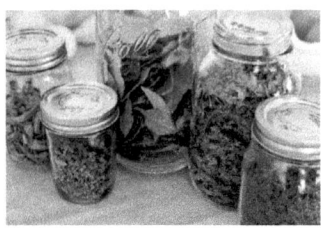

If you have a garden you could easily grow your own medicinal herbs, from plants that you can buy at the local nurseries or from special suppliers of plant seeds. You can even grow many of them in pots on your window sill or in a window box. Some wild plants should be allowed to grow in your garden as they offer great health benefits. The dandelion is one such plant that is constantly being sprayed and killed to make way for our perfect green grass with no dandelions. I myself grow a small area of dandelions in my veggie garden as I like to use the leaves in dandelion tea, and in salads. You also want to make sure that the plants that you are picking are growing in an area where they have not been sprayed with insecticide sprays and other unhealthy chemicals. You should pick plants away from roadsides, gather in real wild places where there is no fear of the plants having been sprayed.

There are certain periods in a plants life when their active constituents are at their peak or optimum level. This is usually when they are just reaching their full growth, you should collect them before they become totally mature. You should thin a patch of plants not totally clearing them so that you are leaving growth for future use in the years to come. When you gather flowers do so when they are fully opened, and dry them quickly away from the sun's direct rays.

If you want to preserve the colour of flowers then you should dry them in the dark. You can spread small flowers on paper and hang the large ones in bunches in an airy dry section. Leaves of the plants are at their best when they have just reached full maturity, nice and fresh, healthy and green. You can gather the leaves or the whole plant above ground just as it is about to flower, spread it on a clean paper, or fine mesh trays or hang them in loose bunches.

Make sure to hang the bunches away from sunlight and in area where the air is able to circulate. You should turn and separate the bunches frequently. The best time to collect plant roots is in the Spring of Autumn. You will need to clean the soil off them and slice them finely for drying by sunlight or in an oven. You should split large roots lengthwise before you chop them.

Plants that contain volatile oils need to be collected in the late afternoon on a sunny day. When drying them do not expose them to heat. You can spread them out and turn them frequently or tie up in loose bunches.

Make sure you are careful when storing plants that are Aromatic plants as the volatile oils they have in them can be absorbed by plastic, making the plant much less useful. You may be able to obtain some good dried herbs from your local health food store. You can find all kinds of herbal teas, compounds and tablets at health food stores that can help in developing a treatment for what ails you. There are formulas that you can purchase at health foods stores that have been made up by herbal practitioners for certain common ailments. There is also many herbal remedies that are prepared by using infusions, salves, or decoctions.

Chapter 2. DIY Salves

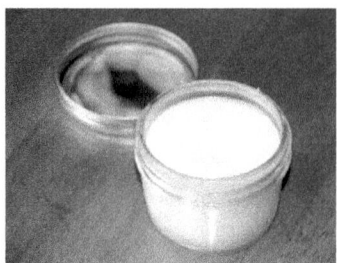

Making salves is not really that hard it basically involves heating up oil, adding beeswax or a vegetable-based wax such as carnuba or candelilla wax, then allowing it to harden into a "balm" pouring it out into jars. When preparing your salve only use herbal oils that have a high smoke point.

To Make Salves You will need:

- one cup of oil either coconut oil or olive oil

- equal parts of dried herbs

- one ounce of beeswax, shaved or vegetable-based wax such as carnuba or candelilla wax

- cheesecloth

- jars to put salve in either in dark glass jars or tin containers.

- Essential oils as needed these are optional

Making Herbal Oil Infusion:

Take a large pot and fill it with one-quarter of water, then place a smaller pot inside of it. Add your oil and herbs to small pot, make sure not to get water in your small pot. Bring to a boil then turn down to simmer for 60 minutes. Place cheesecloth over a funnel and pour herbal infusion over the cheesecloth, squeeze out the remaining oil. You can choose to compost cheesecloth and herbs or if you use coconut oil you can wrap it up and tie and string or rubber band around it and use it in your bath as a nice moisturizer. In a small pan put in the shaved beeswax and then pour over it the infused herbal oil, heat on low and blend together. Pour mixture into jars or containers. When you use less beeswax you will get a creamier salve for a harder one use more beeswax. Using glass or stainless steel containers will work the best for holding your salve.

Ingredients Used for Specific Properties in Salve Recipes:

- Vitamin E is an antioxidant that is great at helping with the healing process. It is also a natural preservative.

- Shea butter has pain relieving properties and is an anti-inflammatory and will also help with dry skin.

- Macadamia nut oil is very good for burns, bedsores, fragile skin, chapped skin and extremely dry skin.

- Avocado oil is a good base for salves that you are using to treat acne, burns, skin problems, it is very good to use on sensitive skin.

- Sweet Almond oil is a great base to use in salves for muscular aches, inflammation, irritation, itching and pains it is a superior emollient.

- Olive oil makes a very greasy oil, it is a wonderful moisture barrier that to get the best results you should use it in combination with other oils.

- Coconut oil is anti-fungal and anti-bacterial, it is great for diaper rash, and to be used in salves for burns, face and hemorrhoids

List of Different Herbs to Make Salves:

1. ***Arnica Flowers.*** These can help you to treat physical trauma, strains, bruises, and muscle pain. Use right after you have developed strain or discomfort.

2. ***St. John's Wort.*** Good to help treat minor wounds, cuts, nerve support, and minor burns.

3. Plaintain leaf. Helps to speed up recovery process, will relieve poison ivy, itching, blisters, damaged skin and stings.

4. Oregon Grape Root. This works great as a skin disinfectant.

5. Nettle Leaf. Works well for many skin irritations.

6. Myrrh Gum Powder. Used for cuts, scrapes, and abrasions.

7. Lavender flowers. Lavender flowers is very soothing herb, has calming effect, relieves pain, offers healing properties for minor wounds.

8. Goldenseal leaf/root. Helps heal minor wounds and skin irritations.

9. Echinea herb/root. Very beneficial for stings, insect bites and sores.

10. Country leaf/root. This will help to relieve pain, swelling, and it supports muscle, bone and cartilages. Helps heal a wide variety of conditions.

11. Chickweed. This is very soothing and will help with the healing of minor burns, and other skin conditions.

12. Chamomile flowers. Good at healing minor cuts and abrasions.

13. Cayenne Pepper. Great for sore muscles, and will alleviate pain and itching.

14. Calendula flowers. Is useful for a wide variety of skin irritations such as rashes, scrapes, wounds, and is good for sensitive skin and babies.

15. Burdock. Works well to help heal skin infections.

Now you are all set to make your own DIY salves using the above herbs and the basic salve formula, and you can make a custom made salve work for the specific condition that you need it for.

Salve Recipes:

1. First Aid Salve

Ingredients:

- one part Calendula oil
- one part comfrey oil
- one part Goldenseal oil
- one drop of lavender essential oil
- one eighth of a teaspoon of tea tree oil
- 800IU vitamin E

Directions:

Use this like you would any basic herbal salve. This is a salve that is anti-bacterial, anti-fungal and will promote rapid healing. It is good to use on cuts, scrapes, and infections.

2. *Lip Salve*

Ingredients:

- one part lavender essential oil
- one part rose essential oil
- one part comfrey oil
- 800IU vitamin E

Use with Lanolin as it helps to heal dry cracked skin, and will keep it nice, soft and subtle. Coconut oil works well in this salve.

3. *Salve of Gardeners*

Ingredients:

- two parts plantain oil
- one part vitamin E oil
- three parts St. John's Wort oil
- three parts of Calendula oil
- three parts of comfrey oil

You can use any salve base. Rub this onto your dry skin, calluses, and psoriasis.

4. Burn Salve

Ingredients:

- 10 drops of lavender essential oil
- one capsule of vitamin E
- one part coconut oil
- one part beeswax, grated
- four parts of Shea butter

Apply to the burn this will help with healing of the skin.

5. Hemorrhoid Salve

Ingredients:

- one part of comfrey oil
- one part of Calendula oil
- one part of nettle leaf oil
- 800IU vitamin E
- one part of Lavender essential oil
- two teaspoons of powdered myrrh

Use this with any salve base.

6. Chest Rub Salve

Ingredients:

- one part thyme essential oil
- one part rosemary essential oil
- one part peppermint (not essential oil, homemade infusion)
- half a teaspoon of eucalyptus essential oil
- half a teaspoon of camphor essential oil

Use recipe with any salve base.

7. Diaper Rash Salve

Ingredients:

- one part lavender essential oil
- one part Calendula oil
- one part comfrey oil
- 800IU vitamin E

Use this recipe with a lanolin base.

8. Black Drawing Salve

The recipe for black drawing salve has not really changed in hundreds of years. The Native Americans, use it to help to draw out toxins and foreign bodies while trying to promote healing.

Ingredients:

- one tablespoon of manuka honey
- one tablespoon of olive oil
- one tablespoon vitamin E oil
- two tablespoons of beeswax
- 15 drops of lavender essential oil
- three tablespoons of rhassoul clay
- three tablespoons of Shea butter
- two tablespoons of activated charcoal powder
- two tablespoons of extra virgin organic coconut oil

Directions:

You will need a spoon, candy thermometer, a two-quart saucepan, cheese grater, two two-ounce jars and bowls. Now put the activated charcoal into a bowl and set it aside. Grate your beeswax and place into a bowl and set aside. In the saucepan put in Shea butter, coconut oil, and beeswax. Heat this mixture to about 180° degrees. Keep this temperature steady for about 15 minutes, use the candy thermometer as a guide tool. Remove the mixture from the stove. Add in the remaining ingredients except for the essential oil. Stir until well blended. Add in the lavender essential oil after your mixture has cooled for 15 minutes. Put your salve into clean glass jars and cover tightly. Store your salve in a cool and dark location in order to preserve its freshness.

9. Wasp Sting Salve

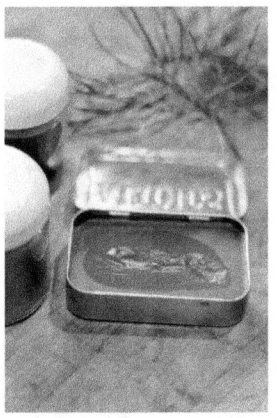

Ingredients:

- one part baking soda
- one part vinegar
- Aloe vera gel
- plantain

Mix plantain (common weed) with warm water and mince it along with baking soda and vinegar and Aloe vera gel then apply directly to the wound.

10. Healing Skin Salve

Ingredients:

- one quarter of a cup of dried marigold flowers
- two tea cups cold-pressed extra virgin olive oil
- half a tea cup of beeswax, melted
- five drops of lavender essential oil
- five drops of tea tree essential oil
- two tablespoons of Shea butter
- three tablespoons of coconut butter

Directions:

In a pot mix your coconut butter, olive oil, dried herbs, simmer in a double boiler on low hear for 3-4 hours, make sure that your water does not all steam away. Remove from heat and strain your herbs out of oil make sure to remove all of the particles of the herbs from oil. Melt the beeswax and Shea butter in double broiler, mix with olive oil and coconut as soon as they are melted. Mix well until you have a nice smooth mixture. Add in your tea tree and lavender essential oils. Pour your mixture into jars with lids. Wait for mixture to harden before you seal the jars with their lids. This salve has no artificial fragrances or preservatives but in its ingredients there are natural preservatives that will keep it from going bad for 1-2 years.

11. *Classic Burn Salve*

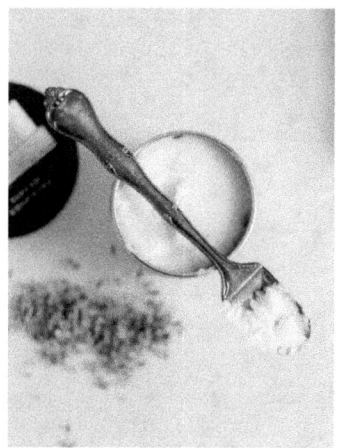

Ingredients:

- one part olive oil
- beeswax, grated
- one part St. John's Wort flowers
- one part comfrey root
- one part comfrey leaves
- one part Calendula flowers

Directions:

In a double broiler place in top pot your comfrey leaves and root, St. John's Wort flowers, Calendula flowers, and olive oil, fill the bottom pot half full of water bring to a low boil. Let the oil simmer for about one hour, check often to make sure it is not overheating, and that you still have water in the bottom pot. Strain the oil and put it into a pan along with beeswax—one quarter of a cup per cup of infused oil. Heat on low, once the beeswax has totally melted remove from heat. You can change the consistency of your salve by adding more oil or more beeswax. If it is too oily add more beeswax, if it is too hard add more oil. Once you have reached the consistency that you desire put your salve into clean glass jars. You can store it up to seven months.

12. DIY Sleep Salve

Ingredients:

- one tablespoon of beeswax pellets
- five tablespoons of almond oil
- three tablespoons of cocoa butter
- 20 drops of rose essential oil
- 20 drops of orange essential oil
- 20 drops of lavender essential oil
- half a vanilla bean, scraped
- one tablespoon of brewed chamomile tea

Directions:

In a saucepan combine all of your ingredients except for the essential oils, heat over low-heat and gently warm just enough for the solids to melt. Remove mixture from heat and stir well, allow to cool. Add in your essential oils and mix again. Pour into glass jars and allow to cool for another 15 minutes, then seal on the lids and store in a cool and dark place. You will be able to keep this salve up to 8 months but it is best to use sooner than later as the scent will diminish over time.

13. *Lanolin Foot Salve*

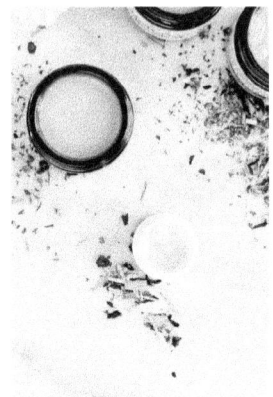

Ingredients:

- four ounces of pure lanolin
- five drops of rosemary essential oil
- five drops of tea tree essential oil
- five drops of needle essential oil
- five drops of lavender essential oil
- five drops of vitamin E oil
- one quarter of a teaspoon of sea buckthorn oil
- half a teaspoon of neem oil
- five tablespoons of cocoa butter
- three tablespoons of Shea butter
- one and a half tablespoons of olive oil infused with Calendula flowers, plantain leaves and comfrey leaves
- one tablespoon of beeswax

Directions:

Start by making your herb infused olive oil. You will need to gather your calendula flowers, plantain leaves, comfrey leaves and place them inside a mason jar. Cover the herbs with oil and then tightly close the lid of jar. Keep in a cool dark place turning occasionally for six weeks. You can also choose a faster approach by placing the mason jar full of herbs and oil into a pot filled about two-thirds full of water. Heat on the stove over low-heat for four hours.

Remove from heat and allow jar to cool. Strain your oil removing the herbs then put it back into jar. Now you are ready to make your foot salve. In a double broiler place your beeswax and cocoa butter into it over low heat. Once they are half-way melted add in the Shea butter and lanolin and continue to heat until all contents are completely melted. Stir to mix contents. Add in the infused oil and mix. Add in the remaining ingredients and mix well then add to glass jars allow to cool for twenty minutes then seal on lids tightly and keep in cool dark place.

14. *Chamomile & Rose Calming Salve*

Ingredients:

- four tablespoons of almond oil
- two tablespoons of beeswax, shaved
- two tablespoons of dried chamomile
- four drops of rose essential oil

Directions:

In a double broiler add water to bottom pot about half full, add in top pot dried chamomile, and almond oil cook on simmer for four hours. Strain the oil removing the herbs when it has cooled. Add infused oil to pan along with beeswax over low heat, mix well and remove once beeswax has melted. Add in the essential oil and mix again. Pour into glass jar and allow to cool for twenty minutes then seal tightly with lid and keep in dark cool place.

15. *Chickweed Salve*

Ingredients:

- two large handfuls of chickweed
- one and a half cups of almond oil
- one ounce of beeswax, shaved
- 30 drops of lavender essential oil

Directions:

Chop up your fresh chickweed finely and lay out on a cookie sheet for 24 hours. The next day add your chickweed to your almond oil and mix well. Put them into blender and blend for about 20 seconds.

Now take this mix and place it in a double broiler in the top pot with the bottom pot filled about half-full or less of water. Bring the water to a boil then reduce to simmer, stirring occasionally. Remove from heat and allow to cool for several hours. Repeat this process. Do not let the oil get so hot that it smokes. The oil will take on a green colour when it has infused with the chickweed. Strain the chickweed using a cheesecloth from the oil. Take the oil and add to a pan with the beeswax and melt over low heat. Remove from heat and add the lavender essential oil and mix well. Pour into tin containers or glass jars. Let sit for twenty minutes with lid off then secure on the lid and keep in a cool and dark place.

Chapter 3. Additional Herbal Remedies for Common Ailments

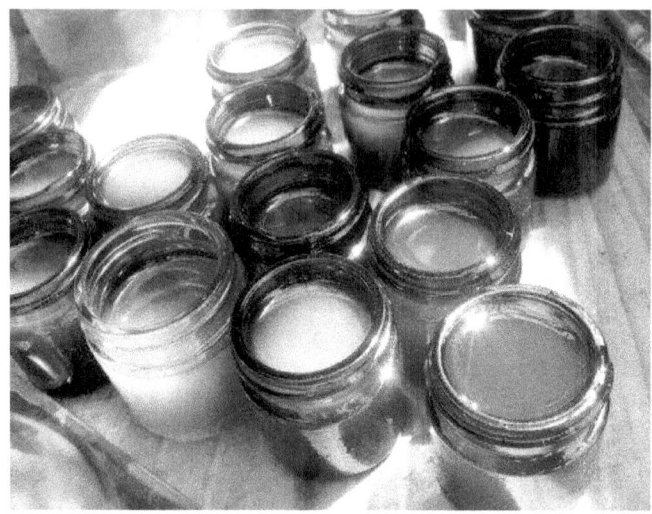

In this chapter we will take a look into various common ailments and the herbal remedies used to treat them.

1. Abscesses, Boils, Carbuncles

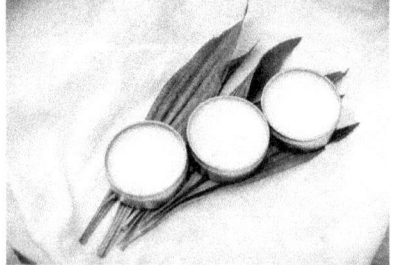

When you have an abscess this is a sign that the body is trying to dispose of toxic waste, it is good to let it come to the point where it bursts to discharge its contents from within the body. You may help this process by covering with a herbal salve or poultice, this will be changed at regular intervals, and then bathing when the salve is changed. You can boil some nettles in water, just enough to cover them. Apply salve hot and change it every eight hours. You can also use crushed fenugreek seeds that you mix to a paste with hot milk, spread on a cotton fabric and fix this salve firmly over the abscess and this will help to draw out the abscess contents. A salve of castor oil can also work.

A salve can be made with powdered slippery elm with a pinch of capsicum, make into a paste using boiled water. Apply this to lint on smooth side and place on the abscess, change every twenty-four hours. Do not try to squeeze the abscess wait until it is ready to burst. Keep applying slippery elm this will clear the abscess and will encourage healing. If you find you are having recurring boils or abscesses you should give some attention to your diet. Add more veggies and fruits to your daily diet. Drink herbal teas such as fumitory and burdock root. Add to boiling water then allow to cool then strain, take a glass full three or four times a day.

2. Acidity

An excessive production of the digestive acids is known as Hyperacidity in the stomach, this can often be connected to emotional stress or mental stress. The best herb when tending to nervous disorders is meadowsweet. Infuse one ounce in a pint of boiling water; take three cups of this a day and it will help correct the acidity problem. You may also combine equal amounts of meadowsweet, dandelion root and centaury herb, one ounce of the mixed herbs to one pint of boiled water. Take a glass after your meals. Chamomile and peppermint tea are useful as well. You should add plenty of alkaline foods to your diet such as veggies and fruits such as apples and pears. There is enzymes in pineapple that aid in the digestion, use pineapple juice diluted in warm water equal parts about an hour after your meals.

3. Acne

This skin problem occurs when the sebaceous glands of the skin become blocked and inflamed, it is often caused by glandular changes which takes place during adolescence, that is worsened by a poor diet. If a person has nervous tension this could cause the condition to worsen. There are a number of remedies for this condition that herbal practitioners offer. They will include dandelion root, burdock root, echinacea, and red clover. These are all mixed in equal quantities with a one ounce mixture that is simmered gently for fifteen minutes in one and a half pints of water; then cooled down. This mixture should be taken three to four times a day. You may want to include remedies for the lymph glands and liver such as blue flag root, barberry bark, chickweed, and poke root.

Try to make yourself more relaxed using tisanes of chamomile flowers or lime blossoms along with an infusion of lavender can be taken as a calming remedy. It can also be used on the skin. Add a handful of stalks that are fresh, to half an ounce of boiling water, cover and infuse for ten minutes. Strain and have a small teacup in the morning and at bedtime. If you have oily skin using cream of marigold flowers is good. Using an infusion of elder flowers is known to be a good skin tonic. To sooth and heal skin you can infuse comfrey leaves for ten minutes then strain and cool then pat onto skin. Avoid using harsh perfumed soaps and do not squeeze spots, keep clean. Try not to use makeup. Add to your diet plenty of raw veggies such as parsley, watercress, dandelion leaves, grated carrot. For good healthy skin you should make sure that you are getting plenty of Vitamin B complex, vitamin A, and E to keep your skin healthy.

4, Allergies

Many of us have hypersensitivity to a wide assortment of substances such as pollen, dust, cat or dog dander, wheat, milk, perfumes, and cheese. These are just a few of a long list of things that people many people are allergic to. Common allergic reactions are watery eyes, recurrent colds, skin rashes, fatigue, diarrhoea, hyperactivity, mood swings, irritability and poor sleep. Part of the answer is to avoid offending foods to help overcome hypersensitivity a herbal practitioner will offer remedies that will improve function of your kidneys, liver and digestion. Using centaury, dandelion root, vervain and fumitory for your liver, gentian root and calumba root to help stimulate your digestion. There are a number of remedies that will be applied according to the individual's needs. You can use chamomile or peppermint tea to help but the allergic condition needs to be addressed comprehensively. Eating a good diet including herbal teas, can overcome your allergic state. It is often recommended that a raw-food diet is best.

Staying away from processed foods and replacing with a high amount of raw salads will have a beneficial effect.

5. Anaemia

In the case of anaemia it could be caused by a lack of haemoglobin (this is the red pigment in blood which carries iron) or it could be a reduction in the number of red blood cells in the bloodstream. Your red blood cells carry oxygen from your lungs to all the other parts of your body. When the oxygen is combined with iron it forms haemoglobin; if you are lacking in either of these it could lead to debility, faster heartbeat, headaches, and a general feeling of malaise. It can also be caused by blood loss such as a haemorrhage or heavy menstruation, it could be secondary due to another illness, it may be failure of bone marrow to produce new cells, or the body is not getting enough iron from food. A herbal practitioner will give remedies that are going to help with digestion and with offering herbal alternatives that can help improve the quality of blood.

A drink that can help with this ailment is made from equal parts of nettles, dandelion roots, vervain, marigold flowers, and comfrey leaves. Using one ounce of each allow them to stand in three pints of cold water for one hour, then bring mixture to boil, keep at boiling point for at least five minutes, then bring to simmer for two minutes. Strain mixture when it has cooled, and take a glassful half an hour before each meal. You can also make a tea of hops or bog bean take a glassful of this after each meal, this will help your body to assimilate iron.

Herbs that contain iron are blackberries, nettles, alfalfa, parsley, chickweed, watercress, and elderberries. If elderberries are taken in large quantities they will act like a laxative. Eat lots of foods such as onions, green leafy veggies, prunes, figs, molasses, brown rice, oats, whole grains, almonds, sunflower seeds, lentils and soya beans. Soya beans will provide you with iron, calcium and other important minerals.

6. Arthritis

Arthritis is a form of rheumatism that the joints become inflamed, affecting cartilages, ligaments and other tissues controlling joint movement, and the bones themselves. There are two main types: rheumatoid arthritis, this is a systematic disease that effects many joints throughout the body, and osteo-arthritis that occurs in weight-bearing joints. Both types may be present at the same time, it also occurs in other forms. A herbal practitioner will use various herbs when treating arthritis, one of the best herbs in treating this condition is meadowsweet, used for its antacid and sedative properties. To reduce the uric acid level corn silk is used, as is gravel root, prickly ash is often added to help improve circulation. Bogbean, burdock root, sarsaparilla, black cohosh, and celery seed are combined with quantities being varied. You can get tablets one that is a must to get would be celery seed tablets. Other products that you might also try are Robert's Prickly Ash Compound, or devil's claw tablets.

Ways that you can help yourself is to have a diet that offers good nutrition, vitamin therapy, exercise, good posture, and having a good positive mental approach. Often those that suffer from arthritis will have low levels of vitamins C, B complex and E. Often drugs that treat arthritis deplete the body of its vitamins, especially vitamins C and B. Taking vitamin C will help in building strong collagen tissue around your joints.

Your diet should include lots of celery, fresh green veggies, parsley, sunflower and sesame seeds, whole grains and homemade veggie soups. Avoid sugars, starches, animal fats, red meat, and alcohol as much as possible. It is also best to avoid citrus fruits, rhubarb, gooseberries, and plums, as many people that suffer from arthritis experience aggravation of pain after they have eaten these kinds of foods. You can find relief by taking a teaspoon of apple cider vinegar in warm water with some honey to add some flavour. You can either take this first thing in the morning or just before meals to help correct deficient production of digestive acids. It is important to exercise to keep your joints mobile.

It is best to avoid tea and coffee replace these with celery seed tea or parsley tea, add a teaspoon of either in a cup of boiling water, cover, cool then strain.

7. Asthma

Under activity of the adrenal glands is what is associated with asthma, as well as sluggish function of the kidneys and also irritability of the nervous system. Asthma sufferers should avoid large intake of milk and sugary foods, as they can aggravate the problem. A herbal practitioner will offer a combination of expectorants to help clear the lungs—these would include coltsfoot, mullein, hyssop, mallow, comfrey, grindelia, and also garlic. Remedies will be to help offer soothing relief of nervous irritability and sensitivity. Chamomile flowers, skull cap, hops and lime blossom are also useful. A good thing to try would be to take a garlic capsule at night and a herbal tea during the day. This could include equal quantities of hyssop, coltsfoot, comfrey leaves, skull cap, and chamomile, one ounce mixed into one pint of simmered water for five minutes, then strained. Take three glassfuls three times a day for an adult and half of that dose for a child. A hot bath which contains catmint or pine would help at bedtime.

It is important to practice deep slow breathing. An asthma attack can be alleviated by adding hot and cold compresses over the chest or by having a hot foot bath. Also you could try a teaspoon of honey with little slivers of garlic that is steeped in hot water and sipped on slowly will help to relieve attack.

Diet should include lots of raw veggies, salads, onions, green veggies and exclude sugar and milk, flour and fatty fried foods.

8. Backache

If you have strained back muscles they will improve if you rest, warmth and massage. Rub back with herbal oil two or three times a day or liniment. You can prepare a simple oil by using fresh, clean, dry St. John's Wort herb with some olive oil and then gently heating it in a pan until the plant loses its fresh green colour and begins to feel crisp. Allow for mixture to cool and then filter it. There are many herbal practitioners that have formulated there own special oils for dealing with backache, others you can find in health food stores.

Conclusion

I hope that you and your loved ones will benefit from this wonderful collection of healthy natural homemade salve recipes. More and more people are turning away from using synthetic forms of treatments for many ailments. Of course it is still always a good idea to talk to your physician about any changes in treatments that you would like to make. This collection of salves will be great in helping you find comfort and relief from many common skin irritations. I wish you the best of luck in finding the right salve for you to help you to heal what ails you!

Thanks again for downloading my book your support of my work is very important to me. I would love to read a review of my book by you on Amazon—take care and happy healing!

FREE Bonus Reminder

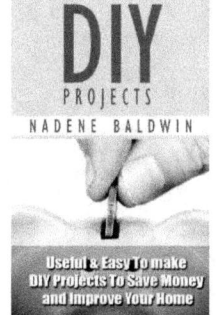

If you have not grabbed it yet, please go ahead and download your special bonus report *"DIY Projects. 13 Useful & Easy To Make DIY Projects To Save Money & Improve Your Home!"*
Simply Click the Button Below

OR **Go to This Page**
http://diyhomecraft.com/free

BONUS #2: More Free & Discounted Books

Do you want to receive more Free & Discounted Books?
We have a mailing list where we send out our new Books when they go free or with a discount on Kindle. Click on the link below to sign up for Free & Discount Book Promotions.
=> Sign Up for Free & Discount Book Promotions <=

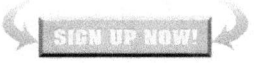

OR Go to this URL

http://zbit.ly/1WBb1Ek

www.ingramcontent.com/pod-product-compliance
Lightning Source LLC
Chambersburg PA
CBHW071321280526
45788CB00004B/1969